Table of Contents

IMPORTANCE OF DIET IN MANAGING GRAVES' DISEASE

1. Impact on Thyroid Function: Certain nutrients play crucial roles in thyroid health, including iodine, selenium, and zinc. While iodine is essential for thyroid hormone synthesis, excessive intake can exacerbate hyperthyroidism in Graves' Disease. Thus, individuals with Graves' Disease are often advised to moderate their iodine intake. Selenium and zinc, on the other hand, are important for regulating thyroid hormone levels and may have anti-inflammatory effects, potentially benefiting individuals with Graves' Disease.

2. Managing Symptoms: Dietary choices can help manage symptoms associated with Graves' Disease, such as weight loss, heart palpitations, and muscle weakness. For instance, consuming small, frequent meals throughout the day can help stabilize blood sugar levels and alleviate symptoms of hyperactivity and fatigue. Additionally, avoiding stimulants like caffeine

and alcohol can help reduce heart palpitations and anxiety.

3. Minimizing Triggers: Some foods may exacerbate symptoms or trigger autoimmune responses in individuals with Graves' Disease. Gluten, for example, has been associated with autoimmune thyroid conditions, and some people with Graves' Disease may benefit from reducing or eliminating gluten-containing foods from their diet. Similarly, certain goitrogenic foods, such as cruciferous vegetables like broccoli and cabbage, may interfere with thyroid hormone synthesis and are best consumed in moderation or cooked to reduce their goitrogenic properties.

4. Supporting Overall Health: A well-balanced diet rich in nutrient-dense foods can support overall health and bolster the immune system, which is particularly important for individuals with autoimmune conditions like Graves' Disease. Emphasizing fruits, vegetables, lean proteins, whole grains, and healthy fats can provide essential vitamins, minerals, antioxidants, and fiber to support optimal immune function and reduce inflammation.

5. Addressing Nutrient Deficiencies: Individuals with Graves' Disease may be at risk of nutrient deficiencies due to malabsorption, medication side effects, or increased nutrient requirements. Working with a healthcare provider or registered dietitian can help identify and address potential deficiencies through dietary modifications or supplementation.

6. Promoting Bone Health: Hyperthyroidism associated with Graves' Disease can increase the risk of osteoporosis due to accelerated bone turnover. Adequate intake of calcium and vitamin D, along with other bone-supportive nutrients like magnesium and vitamin K, can help maintain bone density and reduce the risk of fractures.

7. Personalized Approach: It's essential to recognize that dietary recommendations may vary among individuals with Graves' Disease based on factors such as disease severity, comorbidities, medication regimen, and personal preferences. A personalized approach that takes into account individual needs,

preferences, and lifestyle factors is key to optimizing dietary management.

KEY NUTRIENTS IS ESSENTIAL FOR INDIVIDUALS WITH GRAVES' DISEASE

1. Iodine: While iodine is essential for thyroid hormone synthesis, excessive intake can exacerbate hyperthyroidism in Graves' Disease. Therefore, it's important for individuals with Graves' Disease to moderate their iodine intake. This may involve avoiding iodine-rich foods such as seaweed, iodized salt, and certain seafood, as well as minimizing exposure to iodine-containing supplements and medications.

2. Selenium: Selenium is a trace mineral that plays a crucial role in thyroid function and helps regulate the immune system. Research suggests that selenium supplementation may reduce thyroid antibody levels and improve

thyroid function in individuals with autoimmune thyroid disorders, including Graves' Disease. Good food sources of selenium include Brazil nuts, seafood, lean meats, and whole grains.

3. Zinc: Zinc is another essential mineral involved in thyroid hormone synthesis and immune function. Adequate zinc intake may help support thyroid health and reduce inflammation associated with autoimmune thyroid disorders like Graves' Disease. Food sources of zinc include lean meats, shellfish, legumes, nuts, seeds, and whole grains.

4. Vitamin D: Vitamin D is important for immune function and may play a role in modulating autoimmune responses. Low vitamin D levels have been associated with an increased risk of autoimmune thyroid disorders. Ensuring adequate vitamin D intake through sunlight exposure, fortified foods, or supplements may be beneficial for individuals with Graves' Disease.

5. Vitamin B12: Vitamin B12 is involved in energy metabolism and nervous system function. Some individuals with Graves' Disease may

have impaired absorption of vitamin B12 due to gastrointestinal issues or medication use. Adequate intake of vitamin B12 from dietary sources such as meat, fish, eggs, and fortified foods can help prevent deficiency and support overall health.

6. Omega-3 Fatty Acids: Omega-3 fatty acids have anti-inflammatory properties and may help reduce inflammation associated with autoimmune conditions like Graves' Disease. Including sources of omega-3 fatty acids such as fatty fish (e.g., salmon, mackerel, sardines), flaxseeds, chia seeds, and walnuts in the diet can help promote immune balance and reduce the risk of cardiovascular complications.

7. Antioxidants: Antioxidants such as vitamins C and E, beta-carotene, and polyphenols help neutralize free radicals and reduce oxidative stress, which may contribute to autoimmune dysfunction. Consuming a variety of colorful fruits and vegetables, nuts, seeds, and herbs can provide a range of antioxidants to support immune health and reduce inflammation.

8. Fiber: Adequate fiber intake is important for supporting gut health and promoting regular

bowel movements. Some individuals with Graves' Disease may experience gastrointestinal symptoms or changes in bowel habits, and consuming fiber-rich foods such as fruits, vegetables, whole grains, legumes, and nuts can help alleviate these symptoms and support overall digestive health.

FOODS TO AVOID OR LIMIT

1. Iodine-Rich Foods: Excessive iodine intake can worsen hyperthyroidism in Graves' Disease by stimulating thyroid hormone production. Foods high in iodine include iodized salt, seaweed and kelp products, seafood (such as shrimp, tuna, and cod), and dairy products. While iodine is essential for thyroid health, individuals with Graves' Disease should moderate their intake and avoid excessive consumption of iodine-rich foods.

2. Goitrogenic Foods: Goitrogens are substances that can interfere with thyroid function by inhibiting thyroid hormone synthesis or uptake of iodine. Foods high in goitrogens include

cruciferous vegetables such as broccoli, cabbage, cauliflower, kale, and Brussels sprouts. While these vegetables offer numerous health benefits, they are best consumed in moderation and cooked, as cooking can help deactivate some of the goitrogenic compounds.

3. Gluten: Some individuals with autoimmune thyroid disorders, including Graves' Disease, may have gluten sensitivity or celiac disease. Gluten is a protein found in wheat, barley, rye, and related grains. Research suggests that eliminating gluten from the diet may help reduce inflammation and improve thyroid function in some individuals with autoimmune thyroid conditions. Therefore, individuals with Graves' Disease may benefit from minimizing or eliminating gluten-containing foods from their diet.

4. Caffeine and Stimulants: Caffeine and other stimulants can exacerbate symptoms of hyperthyroidism, such as palpitations, anxiety, and insomnia. Therefore, individuals with Graves' Disease may want to limit their intake of caffeinated beverages like coffee, tea,

energy drinks, and certain sodas. Instead, they can opt for caffeine-free alternatives or herbal teas.

5. Processed and Refined Foods: Processed and refined foods, such as fast food, fried foods, sugary snacks, and refined carbohydrates, offer little nutritional value and may contribute to inflammation and metabolic imbalances. These foods can also lead to fluctuations in blood sugar levels, exacerbating symptoms like fatigue and irritability. Instead, individuals with Graves' Disease should focus on whole, unprocessed foods that are nutrient-dense and support overall health.

6. Alcohol: Alcohol can interfere with thyroid function and may exacerbate symptoms of hyperthyroidism, such as heart palpitations and anxiety. Additionally, alcohol can impair liver function, which is responsible for metabolizing thyroid hormones and medications used to treat Graves' Disease. Therefore, individuals with Graves' Disease may benefit from minimizing their alcohol intake or avoiding it altogether.

7. Soy Products: Soy contains compounds called isoflavones, which are phytoestrogens that may interfere with thyroid hormone synthesis and absorption. While the evidence is mixed, some studies suggest that high soy consumption may negatively affect thyroid function in individuals with autoimmune thyroid disorders. Therefore, individuals with Graves' Disease may choose to limit their intake of soy products, such as tofu, soy milk, and soy-based meat substitutes, especially if they notice adverse effects on their thyroid health.

HEALTHY RECIPES

QUINOA AND ROASTED VEGETABLE PATTY

INGREDIENTS

ROAST VEGETABLES

1. 1 cup pumpkin peeled and cubed
2. 1 cup kumara sweet potato, peeled and cubed
3. 1 large onion diced

4. 1 large red capsicum bell pepper, seeded and diced
5. 1 medium zucchini diced
6. 1 cup button mushrooms stemmed and quartered
7. 1 small eggplant cubed
8. 2 tablespoons coconut oil
9. Salt and ground black pepper
10. 1 sprig of rosemary finely chopped
11. 4 sprigs of thyme leaves removed
12. 1 bunch of fresh parsley finely chopped

QUINOA PATTY

1. 1 cup cooked quinoa both white and black
2. 1 cup cooked brown rice
3. 1/2 c cup basil leaves shredded
4. 1/2 c cup fresh parsley finely chopped
5. 1/4 c cup chives finely chopped
6. Salt and ground black pepper
7. 1/4 c sunflower seeds
8. 1/4 c pumpkin seeds
9. 1/4 c sesame seeds preferably white
10. 1 tablespoon black cumin seeds

INSTRUCTIONS

FOR THE ROASTED VEGETABLES:

1. Preheat the oven to 180°C (350°F).
2. In a large bowl, toss the vegetables with the herbs and oil until they are well coated. Season with salt and pepper.
3. Arrange the vegetables in a single layer on a baking sheet or large roasting dish and bake until they are caramelized and tender, about 25 minutes.

FOR THE QUINOA PATTY:

1. Combine the cooked quinoa and brown rice in a large bowl. Add the fresh basil, parsley and chives.
2. Add the roasted vegetables to the quinoa mixture and blend the ingredients with your hands, slightly mashing them to make the binding for the grains. Season with salt and pepper.

3. Form the mixture into patties of a size you prefer. Generally, a patty of 180g (6 ounces) is sufficient for a meal.
4. Combine the sunflower, pumpkin, sesame and cumin seeds in a small plate. Gently but firmly coat each side of each patty in the seed mixture.
5. Serve the patties cold or at room temperature. You can also heat them in a 150°C (300°F) oven for 20 minutes.

GRAIN-FREE PIZZA

INGREDIENTS

1. 1 cup water
2. 2 cups tapioca flour
3. 1/2 cup coconut flour
4. 2 teaspoon Celtic sea salt
5. 3 tablespoons ghee (or palm shortening for a dairy-free option)

6. 2 large eggs (or 2 gelatin eggs for an egg-free option)
7. 1 1/4 cups shredded mozzarella cheese (omit for dairy-free)

FOR THE SAUCE:

1. 1/2 cup marinara

FOR THE TOPPINGS:

1. Pick which ones you prefer such as cheese, pepperoni, bell peppers, olives, onions, etc.

INSTRUCTIONS

1. Preheat the oven to 425ºF and adjust the rack to the middle position. Line 2 large baking sheets with unbleached parchment paper.
2. Pour the water into a medium saucepan and bring to a simmer. Place the tapioca flour, coconut flour, salt, ghee, eggs and cheese in the bowl of a food processor and pulse to combine. With processor turned on, slowly add the hot water and process until smooth. Let sit for 5 minutes.

3. Spoon the mixture onto the lined baking sheets, placing 2 mounds on each sheet. Using an offset spatula, spread each mound into an 8-inch round (about 1/4" thick). Bake for 12-15 minutes, or until just golden brown on the edges.
4. Spread 2 heaping tablespoons of marinara on each crust. Top with any toppings you want. Bake for 10 minutes, or until the cheese is bubbly and just turning golden brown.

CREAMY ARTICHOKE DIP WITH SPINACH

INGREDIENTS

1. 1 Tablespoon coconut or avocado oil
2. ⅓ cup diced onion
3. 2 cloves garlic, minced
4. 1 cup summer squash, peeled
5. 2/4 cup chicken bone broth
6. 170g drained artichoke hearts
7. 2 Tablespoons nutritional yeast
8. ½ teaspoon ground mace

9. 170g frozen spinach, thawed

INSTRUCTIONS

1. SOFTEN: Add the oil to a pot over a medium heat. Add the diced onion and garlic to the pan. Chop the summer squash into pieces the same size as the diced onion. Add this to the pan and stir to coat with the oil. Cook until the squash is tender, stirring occasionally, so the squash doesn't brown (about 10 minutes)

2. BLEND: Transfer the softened vegetables to a blender and add your chicken broth. Gently squeeze the artichoke hearts to release any excess liquid before you weigh them out. Add the artichoke hearts, nutritional yeast and mace to your blender. Process until you have a thick, smooth 'creamy' sauce.

3. SIMMER: Pour the sauce back into the pot and return to the stovetop at a low heat. Drain the spinach and squeeze out any excess water, then chop finely. Stir the frozen spinach into the sauce and simmer until the dip is warmed through. The dip probably won't need any additional salt because of the artichoke hearts,

but taste now and add salt if you wish. Serve the dip warm and enjoy.

SWEET BEET CHOCOLATE TART

INGREDIENTS

FOR THE CRUST

1. 1/2 cup almonds, ground to meal in food processor
2. 1/2 cup pecans, ground to meal in food processor
3. 1/4 cup ground flax seeds, ground
4. 1 Tbs coconut oil
5. 2 Tbs honey
6. 1/4 cup arrowroot starch (or potato if that's what you have)
7. 1 tsp Vanilla extract
8. 1/4 cup water
9. For the Sweet Beet Chocolate Filling
10. 2 ½ cups grated beets
11. 1/2 cup agave or honey
12. 4 eggs

13. 1/4 cup coconut or grapeseed oil
14. 1/4 cup apple sauce
15. 1 tablespoon vanilla extract
16. ½ cup cocoa

INSTRUCTIONS

FOR THE CRUST

1. Preheat oven to 350.
2. Grind nuts and flax seeds and combine in a mixing bowl.
3. Mix in all remaining ingredients and mix thoroughly.
4. Grease a round pyrex baking dish with coconut oil and press crust mixture evenly around dish (it may help to wet your fingers to keep 'dough' from sticking)- be sure to press it up the sides of the dish as well.
5. Place in oven and bake for about 15-20 minutes until edges start to darken and the crust feels dry.
6. Remove from oven and allow to cool.

FOR THE FILLING

1. Place beets and agave into a pot and bring to a boil. Reduce to simmer for about 15 minutes until beets are soft.
2. In a mixing bowl, mix together eggs, oil, applesauce and vanilla.
3. Puree together beets and agave until smooth texture.
4. Mix beets into wet mixture and then add the cocoa.
5. Mix thoroughly and pour over crust.
6. Return tart to oven and bake for another 35-40 minutes, until cake portion is firm and a tooth pick comes out clean.

PALEO COCONUT CHOCOLATE CAKE

INGREDIENTS

1. 1 1/4 Cup Almond Flour
2. 1 Cup Dark Chocolate Chips or Enjoy Life Chocolate Chips
3. 1/2 Cup Coconut Milk
4. 1/2 Cup Shredded Coconut

5. 1/2 cup Slivered Almonds
6. 2 Eggs
7. 1/2 Tsp Sea Salt
8. 1/2 Tsp Baking Powder
9. Coconut Oil for Grease

INSTRUCTIONS

1. Preheat your oven to 350 Degrees Farenheit
2. Melt your chocolate and coconut milk in a small sauce pan over low heat
3. Once the chocolate is melted, transfer to a mixing bowl or your stand mixer
4. Add in your eggs and mix well
5. Now add in your almond flour, shredded coconut, salt, and baking powder and mix well
6. Grease an 8×8 baking dish with coconut oil
7. Transfer your batter to your baking dish and sprinkle with your slivered almonds and some coconut if you would like
8. Bake in the oven for 25-35 minutes or until a toothpick in the center of the cake comes out clean

CAULIFLOWER WITH GINGER

INGREDIENTS

1. 1 sml/med Cauliflower (head)
2. 4 Tbsp Coconut oil
3. 1 tsp Coriander seeds
4. 1 1/2 Tbsp Ginger (freshly minced)
5. 1 Green chili (seeded and chopped)
6. 1 tsp Turmeric
7. 1/2 tsp Celtic sea salt
8. 2 tsp Lemon Juice (freshly squeezed)
9. 2 Tbsp Coriander (chopped fresh)

INSTRUCTIONS

1. Separate cauliflower into florets, wash well and drain.
2. Heat 3 tablespoons of oil over high heat in a fry pan.
3. When very hot, add the coriander seed and fry for 10 seconds. Add in the ginger, chilies and stir for a couple of seconds. Immediately add turmeric and salt, following with straight away with the cauliflower.

4. Stir rapidly to prevent burning and to distribute the spices.
5. Add 1/4 cup of hot water, reduce the heat to medium – low, cover and cook for 20 to 25 minutes, stirring once or twice.
6. Increase the heat to medium, uncover and stir fry to evaporate remaining moisture and to lightly brown the cauliflower, 5 to 10 minutes stirring carefully.
7. If vegetable look a little dry, stir in the rest of the oil. Add lemon juice and the coriander leaves and toss through.
8. Serve immediately as a side dish.

INSTRUCTIONS

1. 2 tablespoons olive oil (extra virgin)
2. 2 red onions (sliced)
3. 1 tablespoon ginger-garlic paste
4. 1 cup broccoli florets
5. 1/4 cup celery (chopped)
6. 1/4 cup carrots (chopped)
7. Salt (to taste)
8. 1 teaspoon of pepper
9. 1 teaspoon paprika

10. 1 cup of vegetable stock
11. 1/2 teaspoon cumin powder
12. 1/2 cup of coconut milk
13. 1 tablespoon of lemon juice

INGREDIENTS

1. Heat olive oil in a saucepan. Add sliced onion and ginger-garlic paste. Cook for 2 minutes.
2. Now add broccoli, celery, and carrots. Sprinkle salt, pepper, paprika, and cumin powder. Sauté for 5 minutes.
3. Now add vegetable stock and coconut milk. Cook on low heat for 10 minutes. Then take a hand blender and blend the soup.
4. Cook for another 3 minutes. Add lemon juice. Turn off the heat.
5. Serve.

BUTTERNUT SQUASH AND CHICKPEA CHILI

INGREDIENTS

1. 1 large onion, diced

2. 2 ribs celery, chopped
3. 2 cloves garlic, minced
4. 2 15-oz cans chickpeas, drained and rinsed
5. 2 cups butternut squash, diced
6. 2 cups low-sodium vegetable broth
7. 1 15-oz can tomato sauce, no salt added
8. 1 tsp paprika
9. 2 tsp chili powder
10. ½ tsp cumin
11. 2 cups cooked wild rice

DIRECTIONS

1. Place all ingredients except rice in a slow cooker. Stir to evenly combine and cook on high for 4 hours.
2. Serve over wild rice.

BAKED COD

INGREDIENTS

1. 4 cod fillets

2. ground black pepper to taste
3. sea salt to taste
4. 2 tbsp extra virgin olive oil
5. 2 tbsp dijon mustard
6. 2 tbsp lemon juice
7. 1 tbsp parsley
8. 1 clove garlic minced
9. 4 lemon wedge

INSTRUCTIONS

1. Preheat oven to 400 degrees Fahrenheit.
2. Pat the cod dry with a paper towel. Season with salt and pepper.
3. In a small bowl, whisk together the olive oil, Dijon mustard, lemon juice, parsley, and minced garlic to make a sauce. Brush the sauce over the tops of the seasoned cod fillets.
4. Place lemon slices on top of each piece of cod, then bake at 400 degrees for 12-15 minutes, or until the cod is fully cooked.

BROCCOLI SOUP

INGREDIENTS

1. 2 tablespoons olive oil (extra virgin)
2. 2 red onions (sliced)
3. 1 tablespoon ginger-garlic paste
4. 1 cup broccoli florets
5. 1/4 cup celery (chopped)
6. 1/4 cup carrots (chopped)
7. Salt (to taste)
8. 1 teaspoon of pepper
9. 1 teaspoon paprika
10. 1 cup of vegetable stock
11. 1/2 teaspoon cumin powder
12. 1/2 cup of coconut milk
13. 1 tablespoon of lemon juice

INSTRUCTIONS

1. Heat olive oil in a saucepan. Add sliced onion and ginger-garlic paste. Cook for 2 minutes.
2. Now add broccoli, celery, and carrots. Sprinkle salt, pepper, paprika, and cumin powder. Sauté for 5 minutes.

3. Now add vegetable stock and coconut milk. Cook on low heat for 10 minutes. Then take a hand blender and blend the soup.
4. Cook for another 3 minutes. Add lemon juice. Turn off the heat.
5. Serve

CHICKEN APPLE SPINACH HASH

INGREDIENTS

1. 1 Tbsp Coconut oil
2. 1 Lb Organic ground chicken Or turkey, or pork
3. 1 Organic small apple I like Fuji
4. 1 Tbsp Organic maple syrup
5. 2 Tsp Fennel seeds
6. 1 Tsp Sea salt
7. 1 Tsp Paprika
8. 1/2 Tsp Garlic Powder
9. 1/2 Tsp Onion powder
10. 1/2 Tsp Ground sage
11. 1/4 Tsp Red pepper flakes
12. 1/4 Tsp Black pepper

13. 2 Cups Organic baby spinach

INSTRUCTIONS

1. Peel and dice up your apple, cook over medium heat with coconut oil for 2 minutes or until gets soft.
2. Add ground chicken, spices, and maple syrup, mix well.
3. Cook on medium heat for 10-15 min or until chicken is fully cooked, stirring and breaking up large chicken chunks.
4. Add the 2 cups of spinach to the top and cover to allow spinach to wilt. Then mix into the hash, serve and enjoy!

TURKEY APPLE BREAKFAST HASH

INGREDIENTS

1. 1 lb Extra Lean Ground Turkey (or pasture-raised ground chicken)
2. 1 tsp Cinnamon

3. 2 tbsp Poultry Seasoning (2 teaspoons ground
   sage, 1 1/2 teaspoons ground thyme, 1
   teaspoon ground marjoram, 3/4 teaspoon
   ground rosemary, 1/2 teaspoon nutmeg, 1/2
   teaspoon black pepper)
4. 1 tbsp Avocado Oil
5. 1 cup Red Onion (diced)
6. 2 Garlic cloves (minced)
7. 2 cup Brussel Sprouts (trimmed and halved)
8. 2 cup Butternut Squash (peeled and cubed)
9. 2 Orangic Apples (cored and diced)
10. ¼ tsp Sea Salt (to taste)

INSTRUCTIONS

1. Heat a large skillet over medium heat. Add the
   ground turkey, cinnamon, and poultry. Cook for
   5 to 7 minutes, until thoroughly browned,
   breaking up into little pieces as it cooks. Drain
   off the fat, transfer to a bowl and set aside.
2. In the same skillet, heat the oil over medium
   heat. Add the onion and garlic, sauteeing until
   translucent. Next add the brussels sprouts,
   butternut squash, and apples. Cover and cook

for about 10 minutes, stirring occasionally, until all veggies are soft.

3. Add the ground turkey back into the skillet and stir to combine. Season to taste with sea salt. Divide into bowls and enjoy!

FOCACCIA

INGREDIENTS

1. 1 cup + 2 Tablespoons gluten free baking flour blend WITH binder (King Arthur Gluten Free Measure for Measure Flour recommended, see notes)
2. 2 teaspoons gluten free baking powder
3. 1-1/2 teaspoons sugar
4. 1 teaspoon quick rise instant yeast (I like Red Star)
5. 1/2 teaspoon salt
6. 3/4 cup water
7. 1/2 teaspoon apple cider vinegar
8. 1/4 cup + 2 Tablespoons extra virgin olive oil, divided

FOR TOPPING:

1. salt
2. garlic powder
3. Italian seasoning
4. pinch of dried rosemary, crushed between your fingers

DIRECTIONS

1. Move oven rack to the bottom position then preheat oven to 100 degrees using the bread proofing / warming setting. If your oven does not have a bread proofing setting, heat the oven to 100 degrees then turn it off (see notes if your oven doesn't display what temperature it's at while preheating).
2. Add the gluten free flour blend, baking powder, sugar, instant yeast, and salt to the bowl of an electric stand mixer, or a large glass bowl if using a hand-held mixer, then mix on low to combine. Note: if you're using a hand-held mixer, use a whisk to combine the dry ingredients so they don't fly everywhere.

3. Microwave water for 35-40 seconds then stir and take a temperature with an instant read thermometer — we're looking for 110-115 degrees.
4. Pour the water and vinegar into the dry ingredients in the mixing bowl then beat on medium speed until well combined. Let the dough rest for 1 minute. Add 1/4 cup extra virgin olive oil then beat on low speed until just combined. Turn speed up to medium then beat for 1 minute. The dough will be very sticky and similar to cake batter consistency — that's ok!
5. Use a spatula to scrape down the sides of the bowl and give the dough a big stir to ensure the ingredients are well combined. Cover the bowl with a tea towel then place inside the preheated oven and let rise for 30 minutes.
6. After 30 minutes, remove the bowl from the oven, place the oven rack into the center position, then raise the temperature of the oven to 375 degrees.
7. Spray a 9x5" glass loaf pan very well with nonstick spray then add 1 Tablespoon extra virgin olive oil inside and tilt the pan to evenly coat the bottom. Scrape the dough inside then

spread into an even layer. Use the tip of your spatula to dollop the top of the dough to make small peaks which will mimic the dimples usually found on top of focaccia bread after baking (see photos for example). Drizzle remaining Tablespoon extra virgin olive oil on top then sprinkle on salt, garlic powder, Italian seasoning, and crushed rosemary, all to taste.

8. Once the oven has reached 375 degrees, bake bread for 33-35 minutes or until the top of the bread is deeply browned. Avoid under-baking or the bread can be dense and gummy. Let bread rest in the baking pan for 10 minutes before transferring to a cooling rack to cool slightly. Slice then serve while warm.

9. Bread is best baked and eaten on the same day. If there are leftovers, wrap in foil then store on the counter for 1 day. Reheat wrapped in foil in a 350 degree oven until hot, 15-20 minutes.

10. To freeze: Bake focaccia bread then let cool completely. Wrap tightly in foil then place inside a Ziplock freezer bag and freeze. Thaw then bake still wrapped in foil in a 350 degree oven until hot, 15-20 minutes.

INGREDIENTS

1. 350g gluten free plain flour
2. 2 tsp baking powder
3. 300ml natural or plain Greek yoghurt
4. 1 tsp Maldon sea salt
5. 8 sundried tomatoes, finely sliced (optional)
6. 50g green olives, finely sliced (optional)

INSTRUCTIONS

1. Add the flour, baking powder and yoghurt to a large bowl.
2. Mix with a wooden spoon at first to roughly combine then get your hands in there and knead the ingredients until they are properly combined and you are left with a pliable dough. If the mixture is too dry add a little water, if too wet sprinkle with extra flour until you get the consistency pictured below.

3. Add the olives and sundried tomato slices onto the dough and combine to ensure they are evenly distributed throughout. Don't overmix though or your sundried tomatoes with completely meld into the dough (not a bad thing really, as they will still taste great, but visually I prefer to have the red tomato stripes running through the flatbread).

4. Lightly flour a board and rolling pin. Take a sixth of the dough and roll into a ball shape. Flatten it out with the rolling pin until it is around 5mm thick. OR If you are rolling pin-less or in hurry, you can always flatten them with you hands for a more rustic finish. I often do this as it's so quick!

5. Heat a griddle pan over a medium-low flame - oil is optional, these can be dry-fried or simply spritz the pan with a tiny bit of olive oil for a more golden finish. Now pop your raw gluten free flatbread into the pan and allow to cook on each side for around 3-5 minutes. They will rise slightly during cooking, giving a nice light (yet still satisyingly doughy) interior.

6. Repeat steps 4 and 5 until you have a neat little stack of gluten free flatbread and then you are ready to serve!

GLUTEN FREE BREAD

INGREDIENTS

1. 8 g (2 1/2 tsp) active dried yeast
2. 20 g (2 tbsp) superfine/caster sugar
3. 390 g (1 1/2 cups + 2 tbsp) warm water, divided
4. 20 g (1/4 cup) psyllium husk (rough husk form)
5. 130 g (3/4 cup + 3 tbsp) buckwheat flour
6. 100 g (1/2 cup + 3 tbsp) potato starch (NOTE: this is different from potato flour)
7. 90 g (1/2 cup + 2 tbsp) brown rice flour (needs to be very finely ground, "superfine")
8. 10 g (2 tsp) table or sea salt
9. 12 g (2 tsp) apple cider vinegar

INSTRUCTIONS

1. In a small bowl, mix together the yeast, sugar and 150 g (1/2 cup + 2 tbsp) warm water. Set aside for 10 – 15 minutes, or until the mixture starts frothing.

2. In a separate bowl, mix together the psyllium husk and 240 g (1 cup) water. After about 15 – 30 seconds, a gel will form.

3. In a large bowl, mix together the buckwheat flour, potato starch, brown rice flour and salt, until evenly combined.

4. Add the yeast mixture, psyllium gel and apple cider vinegar to the dry ingredients. Knead the dough until smooth and it starts coming away from the bowl, about 5 – 10 minutes. You can knead by hand or using a stand mixer with a dough hook.

5. Transfer the bread to a lightly oiled surface and knead it gently, forming it into a smooth ball. Place the dough into a lightly oiled bowl, seam side down, cover with a damp tea towel and allow to rise in a warm place for about 1 hour or until doubled in size.

6. Once risen, turn the dough out onto a lightly floured surface, and knead it gently while forming it into a tight ball (see post for step-by-

step photos). Flip it seam side down onto a part of the work surface that isn't covered in flour and rotate in place to seal the seams.

7. Place the dough into a 7 inch round proofing basket that you've dusted with some brown rice flour with the seams facing upwards. Cover with a damp tea towel and proof in a warm place for about 1 hour or until doubled in size.

8. While the loaf is proofing, pre-heat the oven to 480 ºF (250 ºC) with a cast iron skillet on the middle rack or a Dutch oven/combo cooker on the lower middle rack. If you're using a skillet, place a baking tray on the bottom rack of the oven.

9. Once the dough has doubled in size, turn it out of the bread basket onto a piece of baking paper and score the top with a pattern of choice (the easiest pattern is a cross, about ¼ – ½ inch deep), using a bread lame or sharp knife. Take the hot cast iron skillet or Dutch oven/combo cooker out of the oven and then transfer the bread along with the baking paper into it.

10. For a skillet or combo cooker, this is easiest by sliding a pizza peel or baking sheet underneath

the baking paper and then using it to slide the bread along with the baking paper gently into the hot skillet/combo cooker. For a Dutch oven, use the sides of the baking paper as handles to transfer the bread into it.

11. If using a skillet: place the skillet in the oven, pour hot water into the bottom baking tray, add 3 – 4 ice cubes around the bread (between the baking/greaseproof paper and the skillet), and close the oven door.

12. If using a Dutch oven/combo cooker: add 3 – 4 ice cubes around the bread (between the baking/greaseproof paper and the walls of the Dutch oven/combo cooker) and close it, then place it into the pre-heated oven.

13. Bake at 480 ºF (250 ºC) with steam for 20 minutes – don't open the Dutch oven or the oven doors during this initial period, as that would allow the steam to escape out of the oven.

14. After the 20 minutes, remove the bottom tray with water from the oven (for cast iron skillet) or uncover the Dutch oven/combo cooker, reduce the oven temperature to 450 ºF (230 ºC), and bake for a further 40 - 50 minutes in a

steam-free environment. The final loaf should be of a deep, dark brown colour. If the loaf starts browning too quickly, cover with a piece of aluminium foil, shiny side up, and continue baking until done.

15. Transfer the loaf onto a wire cooling rack to cool completely.

GLUTEN-FREE SCONES

INGREDIENTS

1. 340 g 2½ cups gluten free self-raising (self-rising) flour
2. 1 tsp gluten-free baking powder
3. 1/4 tsp xanthan gum
4. 85 g 2/3 cup minus 1 tsp butter (use Stork hard margarine if dairy-free)
5. 4 tbsp caster superfine sugar
6. 175 ml ¾ cup minus 1 tsp milk (dairy free if needed)
7. 3 tsp lemon juice
8. 1 1/2 tsp vanilla extract

9. 1 egg to make this vegan, as well as using dairy
   free milk and hard margarine rather than
   butter, you could brush the tops with almond
   milk instead of egg

INSTRUCTIONS

1. Preheat your oven to 220°C/200°C fan/425°F.
   Line a baking sheet with parchment/baking
   paper.
2. Place your gluten free self raising flour, baking
   powder and xanthan gum in a bowl. Chop your
   hard margarine / butter into cubes and add
   that to the flour. Rub it in with your fingers till
   it forms what looks like breadcrumbs.
3. Stir in your caster sugar.
4. Gently warm your milk (I pop it in the
   microwave for about 35 seconds, don't let it
   get really hot, just lukewarm). Then add your
   lemon juice and vanilla extract. Put to one side
   to cool briefly.
5. Place your baking sheet in the oven whilst your
   make your scones. It helps that the baking
   sheet is hot when you place your scones on it.

6. Make a well in the middle of your dry mixture.
    Pour in milk and work it in using a metal spoon.
    Keep working it till it forms a dough (it might
    be a little sticky).
7. Flour (gluten free!) your work surface and your
    hands. Get the dough out of your bowl and fold
    it over a few times to bring the dough together.
    Then bring the dough into a rounded shape
    about 3.5–4.5cm (1¼–1¾in) thick. The taller,
    the better!
8. Using a cutter (about 45–55mm/1¾–2in wide)
    push down into the dough and bring out your
    scones with the cutter. Push them out of the
    cutter and put to one side till you have used up
    all the dough (keep re-rounding the dough).
9. Brush the tops of the scones with beaten egg
    (or with an almond milk wash if you are egg
    free, or have followed this as a vegan recipe
    using dairy free milk and hard margarine).
10. Place the scones onto the hot baking sheet and
    pop them into the oven for about 12-15
    minutes. They should be golden on top and
    have a golden base too ▯
11. Serve up warm with whatever you fancy (jam
    then clotted cream for me!). You can rewarm

them up later, eat them cold, or even freeze them for another day.

INGREDIENTS

1. 1 ripe banana
2. 1 cup spinach leaves
3. 1/2 cup frozen mixed berries
4. 1 tablespoon chia seeds
5. 1/2 cup unsweetened almond milk
6. 1/2 cup Greek yogurt (optional for added protein)
7. 1 teaspoon honey or maple syrup (optional for sweetness)

INSTRUCTIONS

1. Place all ingredients in a blender.
2. Blend until smooth and creamy.
3. Pour into a glass and enjoy immediately.

GLUTEN-FREE OATMEAL WITH BERRIES

INGREDIENTS

1. 1/2 cup gluten-free rolled oats
2. 1 cup water or unsweetened almond milk
3. 1/2 teaspoon cinnamon
4. 1/2 cup mixed berries (such as strawberries, blueberries, raspberries)
5. 1 tablespoon chopped nuts (such as almonds, walnuts, or pecans)
6. 1 tablespoon honey or maple syrup (optional for sweetness)

INSTRUCTIONS

1. In a small saucepan, bring water or almond milk to a boil.
2. Stir in gluten-free oats and cinnamon.
3. Reduce heat to low and simmer, stirring occasionally, for 5-7 minutes or until oats are cooked and creamy.
4. Remove from heat and transfer to a bowl.
5. Top with mixed berries, chopped nuts, and a drizzle of honey or maple syrup, if desired.
6. Serve warm and enjoy.

VEGGIE-PACKED BREAKFAST FRITTATA

INGREDIENTS

1. 6 large eggs
2. 1/4 cup unsweetened almond milk
3. 1 cup diced vegetables (such as bell peppers, spinach, mushrooms, onions)
4. 1/2 cup cherry tomatoes, halved
5. 1/4 cup grated cheese (such as cheddar, feta, or goat cheese)
6. Salt and pepper to taste
7. 1 tablespoon olive oil

INSTRUCTIONS

1. Preheat the oven to 375°F (190°C).
2. In a bowl, whisk together eggs and almond milk. Season with salt and pepper.
3. Heat olive oil in an oven-safe skillet over medium heat.
4. Add diced vegetables and sauté until softened, about 5-7 minutes.
5. Pour egg mixture into the skillet and scatter cherry tomatoes and grated cheese on top.

6. Cook on the stovetop for 3-4 minutes, then transfer the skillet to the preheated oven.
7. Bake for 12-15 minutes or until the frittata is set and the top is golden brown.
8. Remove from the oven and let cool for a few minutes before slicing and serving.

GRILLED SALMON WITH LEMON-DILL SAUCE

INGREDIENTS

1. 2 salmon fillets
2. 2 tablespoons olive oil
3. Salt and pepper to taste
4. 1 lemon, sliced
5. For the Lemon-Dill Sauce:
6. 1/4 cup Greek yogurt
7. 1 tablespoon fresh dill, chopped
8. 1 tablespoon lemon juice
9. 1 teaspoon Dijon mustard
10. Salt and pepper to taste

INSTRUCTIONS

1. Preheat the grill to medium-high heat.
2. Rub salmon fillets with olive oil and season with salt and pepper. Place lemon slices on top of the salmon.
3. Grill salmon for 4-5 minutes per side, or until cooked through and flaky.
4. While the salmon is grilling, prepare the lemon-dill sauce by combining Greek yogurt, fresh dill, lemon juice, Dijon mustard, salt, and pepper in a bowl. Mix well.
5. Serve grilled salmon with lemon-dill sauce on the side. Enjoy with your favorite steamed vegetables or a side salad.

QUINOA SALAD WITH ROASTED VEGETABLES

INGREDIENTS

1. 1 cup quinoa, rinsed
2. 2 cups water or vegetable broth
3. 2 cups mixed vegetables (such as bell peppers, zucchini, cherry tomatoes, red onion)
4. 2 tablespoons olive oil
5. Salt and pepper to taste
6. For the Lemon-Herb Dressing:

7. 2 tablespoons olive oil
8. 2 tablespoons lemon juice
9. 1 tablespoon fresh parsley, chopped
10. 1 tablespoon fresh basil, chopped
11. 1 clove garlic, minced
12. Salt and pepper to taste

INSTRUCTIONS

1. Preheat the oven to 400°F (200°C).
2. In a saucepan, bring water or vegetable broth to a boil. Add quinoa, reduce heat to low, cover, and simmer for 15-20 minutes, or until quinoa is cooked and water is absorbed. Fluff with a fork and let cool.
3. Meanwhile, toss mixed vegetables with olive oil, salt, and pepper. Spread them out on a baking sheet and roast in the preheated oven for 20-25 minutes, or until tender and slightly caramelized.
4. In a small bowl, whisk together olive oil, lemon juice, parsley, basil, garlic, salt, and pepper to make the dressing.

5. In a large bowl, combine cooked quinoa, roasted vegetables, and lemon-herb dressing. Mix well to coat.

6. Serve quinoa salad warm or chilled, garnished with additional fresh herbs if desired.

TURKEY AND VEGETABLE STIR-FRY:

Ingredients:

1. 1 pound turkey breast, thinly sliced

2. 2 tablespoons soy sauce (or tamari for gluten-free option)

3. 1 tablespoon olive oil

4. 2 cups mixed vegetables (such as bell peppers, broccoli, carrots, snap peas)

5. 2 cloves garlic, minced

6. 1 teaspoon fresh ginger, grated

7. Salt and pepper to taste

8. Cooked rice or quinoa for serving

INSTRUCTIONS

1. In a bowl, marinate sliced turkey breast in soy sauce for 15-20 minutes.
2. Heat olive oil in a large skillet or wok over medium-high heat. Add marinated turkey and stir-fry for 5-6 minutes, or until cooked through. Remove from skillet and set aside.
3. In the same skillet, add a bit more olive oil if needed. Add mixed vegetables, garlic, and ginger. Stir-fry for 3-4 minutes, or until vegetables are tender-crisp.
4. Return cooked turkey to the skillet and toss with the vegetables. Season with salt and pepper to taste.
5. Serve turkey and vegetable stir-fry over cooked rice or quinoa. Enjoy hot.

BAKED LEMON HERB CHICKEN

INGREDIENTS

1. 4 boneless, skinless chicken breasts
2. 2 tablespoons olive oil
3. 2 cloves garlic, minced

4. Zest and juice of 1 lemon
5. 1 teaspoon dried oregano
6. 1 teaspoon dried thyme
7. Salt and pepper to taste

INSTRUCTIONS

1. Preheat the oven to 375°F (190°C).
2. In a small bowl, whisk together olive oil, minced garlic, lemon zest, lemon juice, dried oregano, dried thyme, salt, and pepper.
3. Place chicken breasts in a baking dish and pour the lemon herb mixture over them, making sure to coat each piece evenly.
4. Bake in the preheated oven for 25-30 minutes, or until chicken is cooked through and juices run clear.
5. Remove from the oven and let rest for a few minutes before serving. Enjoy with your favorite side dishes, such as roasted vegetables or quinoa pilaf.

TOFU AND VEGETABLE STIR-FRY

INGREDIENTS

1. 1 block (14 ounces) extra-firm tofu, drained and pressed
2. 2 tablespoons soy sauce (or tamari for gluten-free option)
3. 1 tablespoon sesame oil
4. 2 cloves garlic, minced
5. 1 teaspoon fresh ginger, grated
6. 2 cups mixed vegetables (such as bell peppers, broccoli, snap peas, carrots)
7. Cooked brown rice or quinoa for serving
8. Sesame seeds and chopped green onions for garnish

INSTRUCTIONS

1. Cut pressed tofu into cubes.
2. In a bowl, marinate tofu cubes in soy sauce for 15-20 minutes.
3. Heat sesame oil in a large skillet or wok over medium-high heat.
4. Add marinated tofu cubes to the skillet and cook for 5-6 minutes, or until golden brown on all sides. Remove from skillet and set aside.

5. In the same skillet, add a bit more sesame oil if needed. Add minced garlic and grated ginger, and sauté for 1-2 minutes until fragrant.
6. Add mixed vegetables to the skillet and stir-fry for 3-4 minutes, or until tender-crisp.
7. Return cooked tofu to the skillet and toss with the vegetables until heated through.
8. Serve tofu and vegetable stir-fry over cooked brown rice or quinoa. Garnish with sesame seeds and chopped green onions.

STUFFED BELL PEPPERS WITH QUINOA AND VEGETABLES

INGREDIENTS

1. 4 large bell peppers, any color
2. 1 cup cooked quinoa
3. 1 cup mixed vegetables (such as zucchini, carrots, mushrooms, onions)
4. 1 can (15 ounces) black beans, drained and rinsed
5. 1 cup shredded cheese (such as cheddar or mozzarella), divided
6. 1 teaspoon chili powder

7. 1/2 teaspoon cumin

8. Salt and pepper to taste

9. Fresh cilantro, chopped, for garnish

Instructions

1. Preheat the oven to 375°F (190°C). Slice the tops off the bell peppers and remove the seeds and membranes.

2. In a large bowl, combine cooked quinoa, mixed vegetables, black beans, half of the shredded cheese, chili powder, cumin, salt, and pepper.

3. Stuff each bell pepper with the quinoa and vegetable mixture, pressing down gently to pack it in.

4. Place stuffed bell peppers in a baking dish. Sprinkle remaining shredded cheese on top of each pepper.

5. Cover the baking dish with aluminum foil and bake in the preheated oven for 30-35 minutes, or until peppers are tender.

6. Remove from the oven and let cool for a few minutes before serving. Garnish with fresh cilantro before serving.

GARLIC ROASTED BRUSSELS SPROUTS

INGREDIENTS

1. 1 pound Brussels sprouts, trimmed and halved
2. 2 tablespoons olive oil
3. 2 cloves garlic, minced
4. Salt and pepper to taste

INSTRUCTIONS

1. Preheat the oven to 400°F (200°C).
2. In a large bowl, toss Brussels sprouts with olive oil, minced garlic, salt, and pepper until evenly coated.
3. Spread Brussels sprouts in a single layer on a baking sheet lined with parchment paper.
4. Roast in the preheated oven for 20-25 minutes, or until Brussels sprouts are tender and caramelized, stirring halfway through.
5. Remove from the oven and serve hot.

LEMON HERB QUINOA PILAF

INGREDIENTS

1. 1 cup quinoa, rinsed
2. 2 cups vegetable broth
3. Zest and juice of 1 lemon
4. 2 tablespoons fresh parsley, chopped
5. 1 tablespoon fresh thyme leaves
6. Salt and pepper to taste

INSTRUCTIONS

1. In a medium saucepan, bring vegetable broth to a boil.
2. Stir in quinoa, lemon zest, lemon juice, chopped parsley, thyme leaves, salt, and pepper.
3. Reduce heat to low, cover, and simmer for 15-20 minutes, or until quinoa is cooked and liquid is absorbed.
4. Fluff quinoa with a fork and transfer to a serving dish.
5. Garnish with additional fresh herbs if desired and serve warm.

STEAMED BROCCOLI WITH ALMOND BUTTER SAUCE

INGREDIENTS

1. 1 pound broccoli florets
2. 2 tablespoons almond butter
3. 2 tablespoons tamari (or soy sauce)
4. 1 tablespoon rice vinegar
5. 1 tablespoon maple syrup
6. 1 clove garlic, minced
7. 1 teaspoon fresh ginger, grated
8. Water, as needed
9. Sesame seeds for garnish (optional)

INSTRUCTIONS

1. Steam broccoli florets until tender-crisp, about 5-7 minutes.
2. In a small saucepan, whisk together almond butter, tamari, rice vinegar, maple syrup, minced garlic, and grated ginger over medium heat.
3. If the sauce is too thick, thin it out with a little water until desired consistency is reached.
4. Drizzle almond butter sauce over steamed broccoli and toss to coat evenly.
5. Garnish with sesame seeds, if desired, and serve hot.

CONCLUSIONS

Empowering individuals with Graves' Disease to make informed dietary choices and adopt healthy eating habits, the cookbook aims to enhance their quality of life, support symptom management, and promote long-term well-being. It serves as a comprehensive guide for navigating the challenges of meal planning and preparation while living with Graves' Disease, ultimately fostering a positive and nourishing relationship with food.

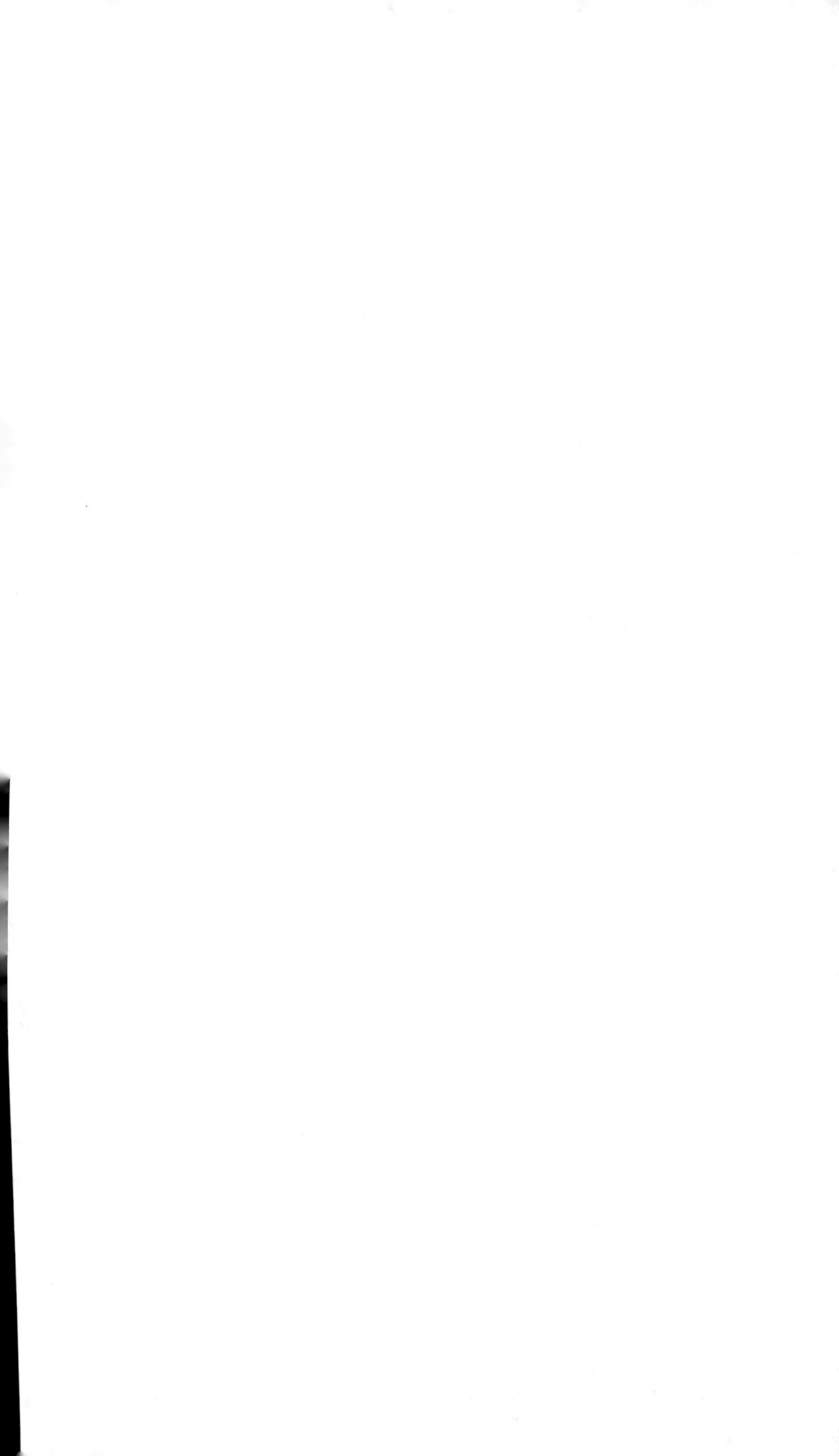